Kawtar Inani

Methotrexate and psoriasis

Kawtar Inani

Methotrexate and psoriasis

ScienciaScripts

Imprint

Any brand names and product names mentioned in this book are subject to trademark, brand or patent protection and are trademarks or registered trademarks of their respective holders. The use of brand names, product names, common names, trade names, product descriptions etc. even without a particular marking in this work is in no way to be construed to mean that such names may be regarded as unrestricted in respect of trademark and brand protection legislation and could thus be used by anyone.

Cover image: www.ingimage.com

This book is a translation from the original published under ISBN 978-3-639-50346-3.

Publisher:
Sciencia Scripts
is a trademark of
Dodo Books Indian Ocean Ltd. and OmniScriptum S.R.L publishing group

120 High Road, East Finchley, London, N2 9ED, United Kingdom
Str. Armeneasca 28/1, office 1, Chisinau MD-2012, Republic of Moldova, Europe
Printed at: see last page
ISBN: 978-620-5-79315-2

METHOTREXATE AND PSORIASIS
Dr. INANI KAWTAR

Table of contents

I.   <u>Introduction</u>

Psoriasis is a chronic inflammatory disease characterized by abnormal activation of the immune system affecting mainly the skin and joints. The onset is early, usually between 20 and 30 years of age. Psoriasis has a major impact on the quality of life of patients. They are confronted with significant personal expenses and social exclusion [1]. The management of psoriasis is a real challenge due to the chronicity of the disease, which requires good compliance, and due to the high cost of treatments and their unavailability.

Methotrexate is an analogue of folic acid, which acts as an antineoplastic and antimetabolic agent by inhibiting cell proliferation. It has been used since the 1950s in several fields, including internal medicine, rheumatology and dermatology. Currently, it is the systemic treatment of reference for moderate to severe cutaneous psoriasis [2,3].

II.   <u>Objectives of the study</u>

> To evaluate the efficacy of methotrexate in the treatment of moderate to severe psoriasis.

> Evaluate the efficacy of methotrexate on the different types and conditions of psoriasis.

> Assessing medication adherence in our patients.

> To assess the clinical and biological tolerance of methotrexate.

> Identify the main side effects encountered in our patients.

III. <u>Materials and Methods</u>

1. <u>Type of study</u>

This was a uni-centric retrospective study with data collection of psoriatic patients followed at the Dermatology Department of the Hassan II University Hospital in Fez. A descriptive and analytical analysis was made.

2. <u>Location of the study</u>

The HASSAN II University Hospital in FES, where patients were recruited during hospital activity or during the weekly specialized psoriasis consultation.

3. <u>Date of the study</u>

Retrospective study conducted in the dermatology department from 2010 to 2014.

4. <u>Study population</u>

4.1 Inclusion Criteria

> Psoriatic patients with HC> 25

> Patients with no absolute contraindications to methotrexate therapy *4.2 exclusion criteria*

> Psoriatic patients with a SC <25%.

> Psoriatic patients with absolute contraindications to methotrexate therapy

> Psoriatic patients who cannot afford regular biological monitoring

5. <u>Methods:</u>

5.1 Sampling

All cases of psoriasis were included and the records of patients treated with MTX were reviewed. A pre-established form was filled out for each patient specifying the type of psoriasis, the indications, the modalities of prescription, monitoring, evolution and side effects.

5.2 Number of participating subjects

200 cases of psoriasis of which 46 were treated with methotrexate.

5.3 Data collection

Data were collected using a pre-designed data collection form that included:

J Socio-epidemiological data:

• Age, gender, phone number, date of onset of psoriasis (how long ago), and prescribed treatments.

J Clinical data

•   Collected through a clinical examination of the skin, mucous membranes, and appendages to determine the type of psoriasis. Body surface area was measured either by the Wallas ruler or by the palm of the hand.

J Therapeutic data: thus were specified:

•   The starting dose of methotrexate, the route of administration, the date treatment was started, the side effects, the cumulative dose, whether or not folic acid was added, and the combination with other local treatments.

J Para-clinical data:

•   Initial and control biological and radiological work-up: CBC, hepatic work-up, renal work-up, albumin, infectious work-up, BHCG, and fibroscans.

J Evolving data: It was considered as :

•   Complete remission: the complete healing of lesions upon discontinuation of methotrexate

•   Improvement: a decrease of the affected body surface by 10%.

5.4   *Operating sheet*

Methotrexate and Psoriasis

> Patient number: ....
> Last and first name ....
> T ....
> Phone number...
> Age ....
> Sex..

Child < 18 years CDCD   Adult 184? years
Adult-?-5C O
> Typedepsoriasis:...

Viigaire   CD   Eiythrodemic CD
Pustuleux   CD   Reverse CD
> Body surface
2? - 50%   O   CD -G-
                >70%O

> Age of onset ....
>   Scalp involvementCD   CD No
>   Reaching к   ч YesCD   No
oral mucosa   'T/
>   Nail damage   CD Yes   CD No
>   Reach   л, Yes   CD No
palino-plantEire
>   Joint involvement CD Yes   CD No
> Breakfast treatment = received .
CD DennocorticoidsCD   Daivonex
v DEivübet
Phototherapy O PUVA   OgiOl
Duration...
> Methotrexate initiation :...
> V c ie d" administration : O ï- -   O VO
> Start date of treatment : ....

	Dose	Check out biological monitoring	Fibroscann	SC PASI	Side effects	Cumulative dose	Folic acid supplementation	Therapeutic association
JO								
3 months								
6 months								
9 months								
12 months								
18 months								
24 months								

5.5 statistical analysis :

Data were entered and validated on an Excel file for analysis using SPSS20 software. For the descriptive analysis: quantitative variables were expressed as mean ± standard deviation and qualitative variables as percentages.

IV. <u>Results</u>

In our series, 46 patients with psoriasis on methotrexate were enrolled.

1. <u>The epidemiological data</u>

1.1 Age

In our sample, patients were divided into three age groups:

A first group whose age was less than 18 years represented 13%, the second group whose age was between 18 and 45 years and whose percentage was 45.7%, and finally people over 45 years represented 41.3%.

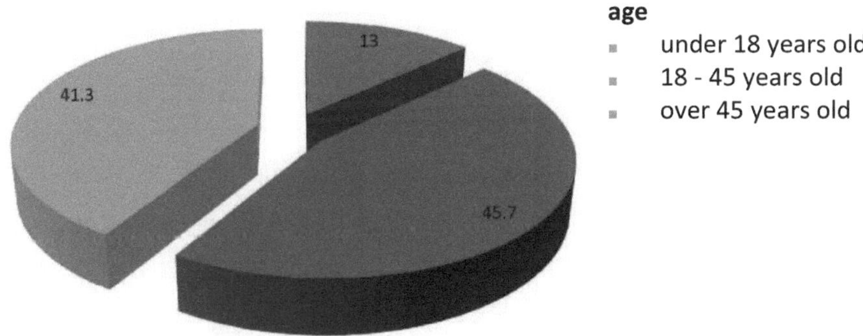

The age of onset was between 18 and 45 years in 50% of cases, compared with 21.7% for the first group and 28.3% for the third group.

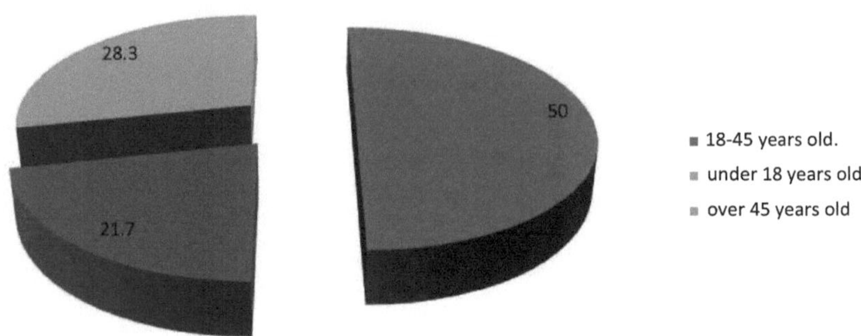

1.2 Gender:

We note a predominance of the male sex with a percentage of 58.7% versus 41.3% with a
gender - F/H ratio of 1.42.

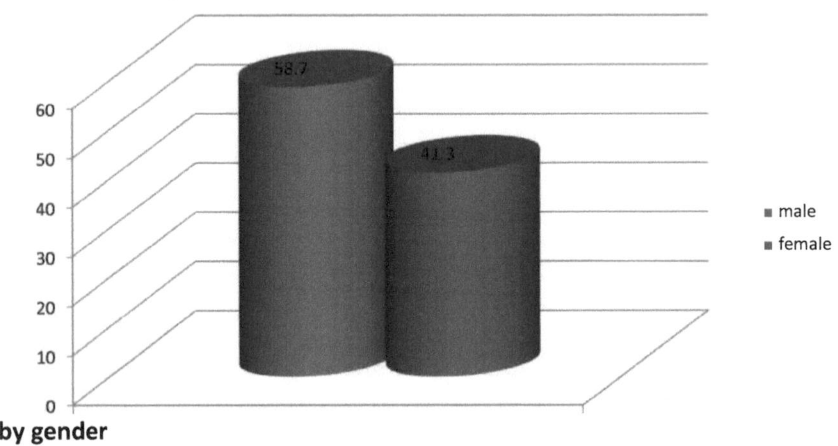

by gender

2.1 Clinical forms

The clinical forms were distributed as follows: psoriasis vulgaris in 35 cases (76.1%), followed by arthropathic psoriasis in 6 cases (13%), erythrodermic psoriasis in 3 cases (6.5%) and psoriatic palmoplantar keratosis in 2 cases (4.3%). Mucosal involvement was found in only 9%, and scalp involvement in 72%.

clinical forms

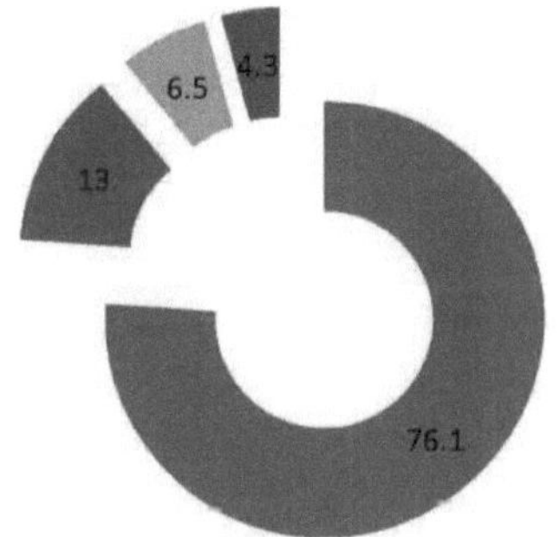

2.2 Body surface area affected

71.7% had a body surface area (BSA) between 25 and 50%, 21.7% had a BSA between 50 and 70%, with only 6.5% having a BSA greater than 70%.

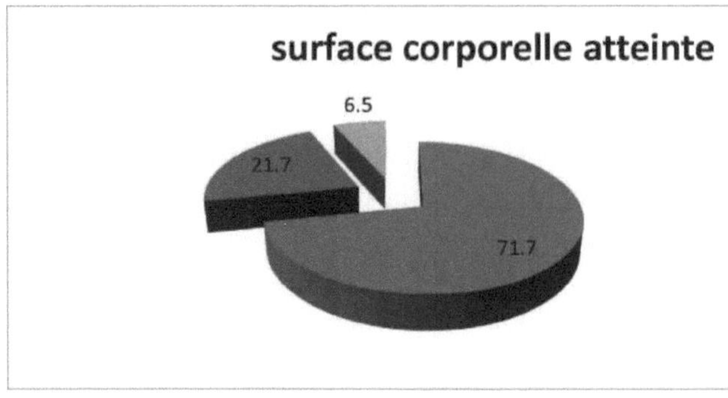

3.1 The weekly dose of methotrexate

The weekly dose ranged from 10 to 30 mg, with a mean dose of 25 mg prescribed in 58.7%.

3.2 Therapeutic associations

MTX was combined with folinic acid and dermocorticoids (DCs) in 82.7% of cases, with DCs alone in 15.2% of cases, and only 2.2% of cases were prescribed MTX in combination with folinic acid and calcipotriol.

therapeutic associations

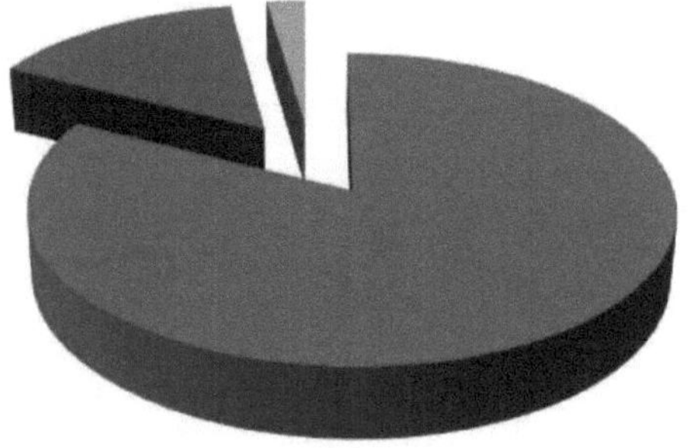

The average duration of treatment was 16.19 months, with a minimum duration of 6 months and a maximum of 24 months.

The evolution was marked by a complete remission in 50% of cases, with an improvement of 21.37% at 6 months, 24.56% at 9 months, 23.18% at 12 months, 26.92% at 18 months and 33.86% at 24 months.

Remission rate

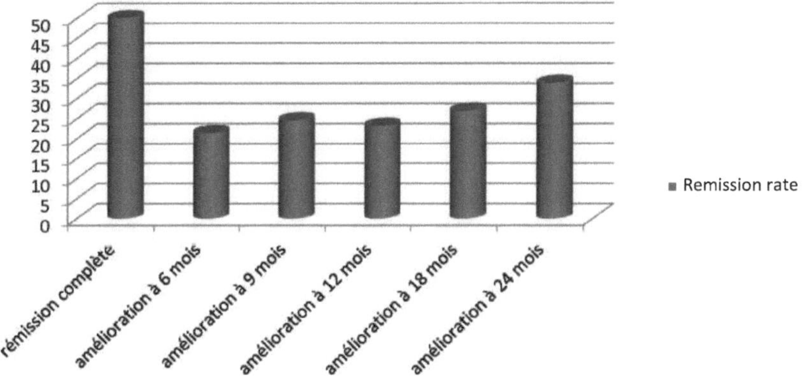

Side effects were mainly digestive intolerance in a 30-year-old man, in whom the dose was reduced, a case of cytolysis in a 55-year-old man and a case of renal failure in a 64-year-old man; for the last two, the treatment was stopped.

V. <u>Discussion</u>

We conducted a retro-prospective study, over a period of 4 years, in which we evaluated the place of methotrexate in the treatment of psoriasis in our Moroccan context. Our study is particular, by the good response of our patients, the rarity of side effects, the good tolerance, thus testifying of our experience in the management of MTX.

1. <u>Psoriasis</u>

1.1   Epidemiology

❖   <u>Prevalence and incidence</u>

Psoriasis is a chronic autoimmune disease that primarily affects the skin and joints. It occurs worldwide and without gender predilection. However, its prevalence varies considerably from region to region. In the United States, psoriasis affects approximately 2% to 4.6% of the population, with an annual incidence ranging from 14 to 60.4 cases per 100,000 population per year [4]. In Morocco, a cross-sectional study was carried out in the Maghreb, involving general practitioners and dermatologists over a period of 2 months, which revealed a prevalence of 1.07/1000 inhabitants, i.e. an annual incidence of 1 to 2% [5].

Psoriasis is extremely rare in some ethnic groups, such as Africans, African Americans, Japanese, Norwegians, Australians, and Alaskans. The prevalence of psoriasis has not changed over time according to epidemiological studies, in contrast to other autoimmune diseases whose prevalence rate has increased [4].

❖   <u>Age</u>

Psoriasis can appear at any age; however, a bimodal distribution is characteristic. The majority of cases, about 75%, have an onset before the age of 40, with a peak between 20 and 30 years. Patients with early onset have a family history of psoriasis, a frequent association with histocompatibility antigen (HLA)-Cw6, and more severe involvement. Those with onset after the age of 40 years usually have a negative family history and a normal Cw6 allele frequency [4].

In a study conducted in our department over one year (November 2011_November 2012) The overall mean age was 37 years with a standard deviation of 17.6 years. [6]

In a study conducted at the Military Hospital of Meknes between January 2006 and December 2012, on the efficacy of methotrexate in the treatment of severe psoriasis, the mean age of patients was 43.4 years. [7]

In our study, 45.7% of the subjects were between 18 and 45 years of age and 41.3% were over 45 years of age, while 13% were children.

Our data are consistent with the literature, as almost half of our patients were younger than 45 years of age with moderate to severe disease.

❖　　　　<u>Sex:</u>

Psoriasis affects the general population without gender predilection, however in the series of the military hospital of Meknes [7], as well as in our series of moderate to severe psoriasis, we found a male predominance, probably related to the delay of consultation of men at the early stage of the disease, or probably to the predisposition of the male sex to severe forms of psoriasis.

1.2　　　pathophysiology

The main features of psoriasis are abnormal proliferation and differentiation of keratinocytes, infiltration of the epidermis by inflammatory cells and vascular changes. The interaction between different cell types such as epidermal cells, cells involved in the immune response (T cells and antigen-presenting cells) and those of the vascular system (endothelial cells) seems to play a role in the pathogenesis of the disease, but the primary defect responsible for this disease remains unidentified.

It is in fact a delayed hypersensitivity reaction (mediated by T lymphocytes) with a two-phase course:

❖　　　**An initial awareness phase:**

Clinically silent, it requires the presence of an as yet unidentified antigen, probably located in the keratinocytes (perhaps in relation to HLA-Cw6) and which would thus give the starting signal to the pathological process. Some authors believe that there are cross-reactions between certain proteins in the keratinocytes (especially keratin) and bacterial (streptococcal M- proteins) or viral antigens [8]. It is possible that infections or traumas themselves induce the production of proinflammatory cytokines (tumor necrosis factor alpha (TNF-a), interferon (IFN)) as well as co-stimulatory and adhesion molecules (CD2/LFA-3, LFA-1:ICAM-1) are required before an activating T-cell response can be initiated [9,10]. This phase takes place in the lymph node.

❖ **A second phase of expression:**

It begins with the activation of T lymphocytes that interact with antigen-presenting cells, which activates the two lymphocyte profiles Th1 and Th17. The inflammatory reaction thus produced is accompanied by the release of a series of pro-inflammatory cytokines (IL-1, IL-6, TNF-a, IFN-g), chemokines (IL-8), growth factors (vascular growth factor), and other substances (e.g., antigen-presenting cells) by both resident and migrating cells (T cells, dendritic cells, macrophages, mast cells, keratinocytes, endothelial cells, neural cells).

growth factors (vascular endothelial growth factor = VEGF) and neuropeptides. Some of these factors increase the proliferative activity of basal layer keratinocytes, while others lead to the recruitment of other proinflammatory cells, in particular neutrophils. At the same time, the activation of endothelial cells results in the expression of adhesion molecules and vasodilation which slows down blood flow, thus allowing extravasation of inflammatory cells [11, 12, 13,14].

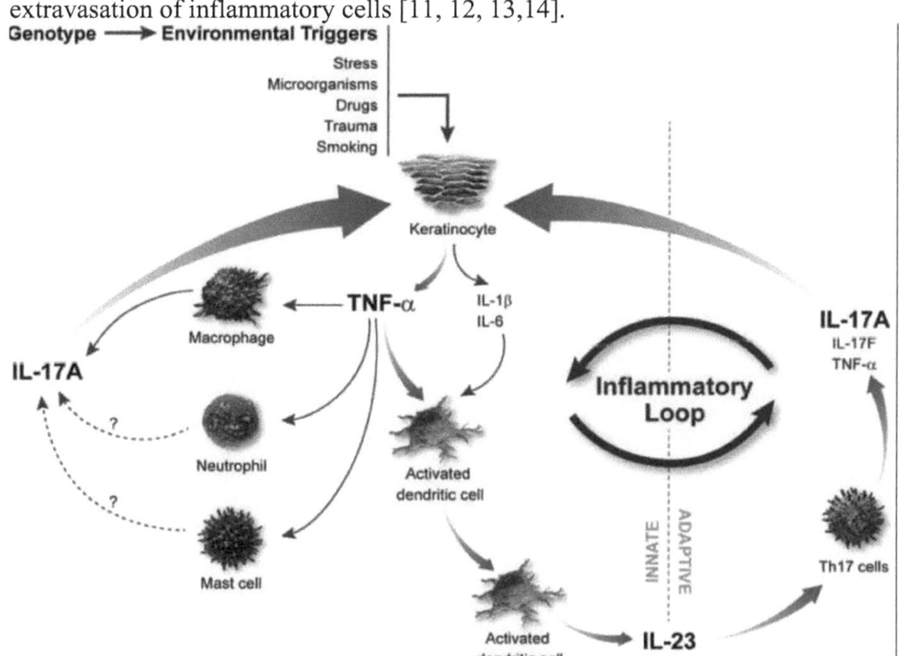

Figure 1: Activation and genesis pathways of psoriasis [15]

Plaque psoriasis or psoriasis vulgaris, the most frequent form, presents clinically as erythematous-squamous plaques, well limited, variable in size, the scales are usually whitish and thick, symmetrically distributed on pressure areas also called bastion areas: elbow, ulnar edge of the forearm, knee, pre-shin regions, lumbosacral region and scalp. [6,16]

This form is also the most frequent in our series with a percentage of 76.1%.

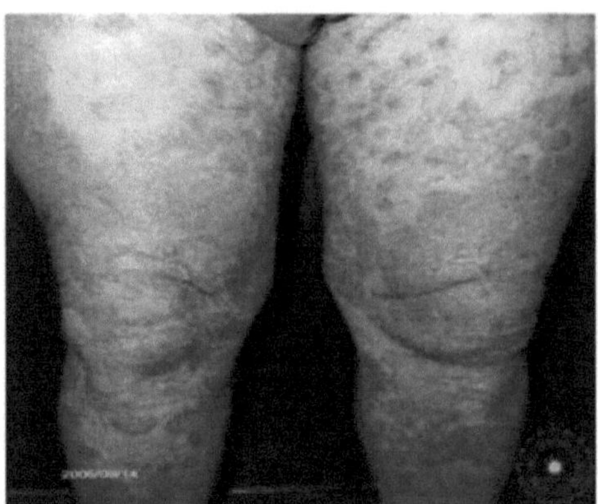

Figure 1: Plaque psoriasis

1.3.2 Guttate psoriasis :

The most frequent form in children and adolescents, it generally occurs following an infectious episode, and takes the form of small erythematous, finely scaly patches of less than 1 cm. [17]

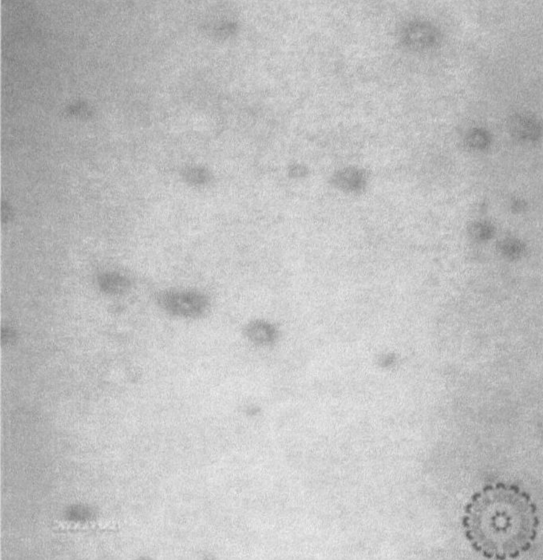

Figure 2: Guttate psoriasis

1.3.3 Psoriasis of the folds :

It presents as a chronic intertrigo, made up of bright red placards, with little or no scaling, with clear contours, all folds can be affected. Its diagnosis remains difficult, in the absence of

remote lesions. [16, 17,18]

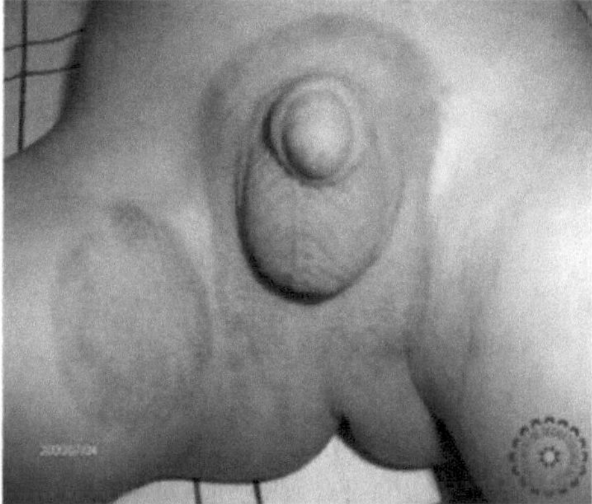

Figure 3: Fold psoriasis

1.3.4 Psoriasis of the scalp :

Scalp involvement is quite often seen in association with skin involvement, rarely isolated. It presents either as erythematous patches covered with dry or oily scales or as a carapace involving the entire scalp. [19]
In our series, scalp involvement was present in 72%.

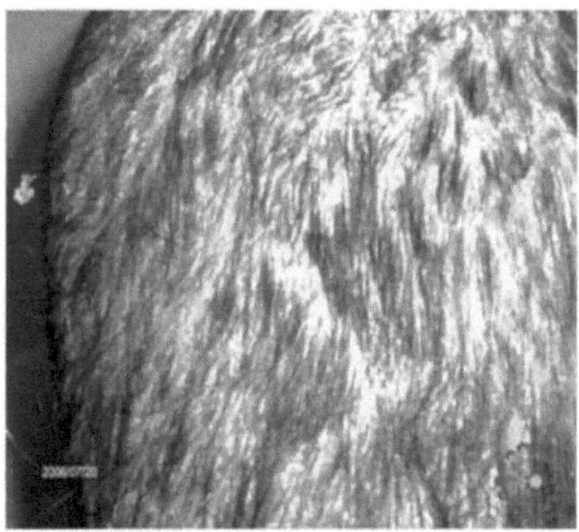

Figure 4 : scalp shell

This form classically presents as keratotic plaques, sometimes fissured, which may evolve into full-blown KPP. [20]

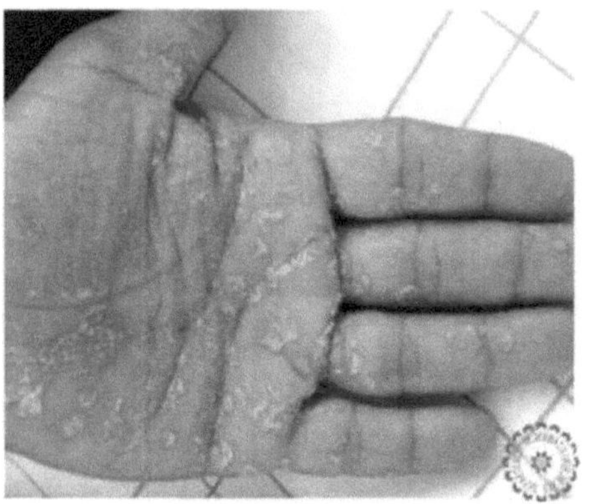

In our study, 2 cases of KPP were treated with methotrexate, i.e. 4.3%.

Figure 5 a and b: palmoplantar psoriasis

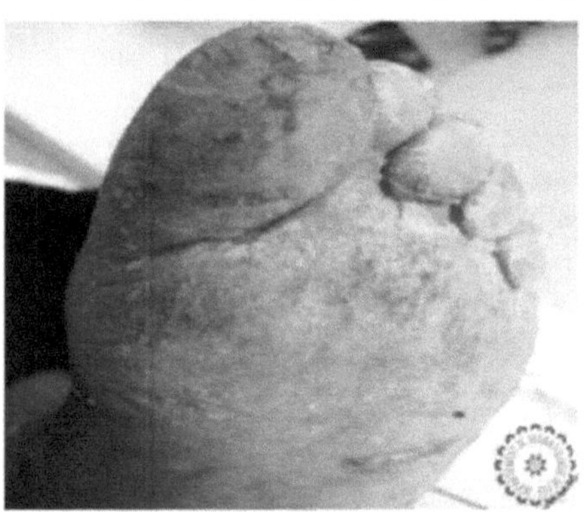

It is associated in 30 to 50% of cases with isolated cutaneous psoriasis; it poses a real diagnostic problem, requiring a nail biopsy. Several aspects can be seen:

Thimble-like appearance, trachyonychia, leukonychia, oil stain, onycholysis, pachyonychia, paronychia, hemorrhages and subungual pustules. [21]
In our series, nail involvement was present in 89.2% with a thimble-like appearance in 43.5%, and pachyonychia in 45.7%, which we could not classify as psoriasis since these patients did not undergo mycological sampling.

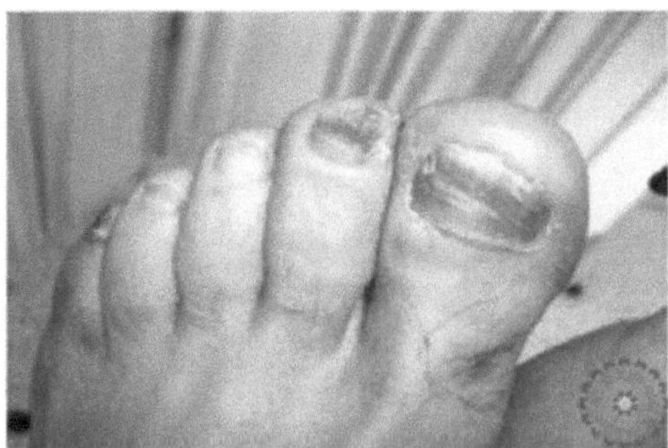

Figure 6: Ungual psoriasis

1.3.7 Pustular psoriasis :

Amicrobial pustulosis, localized forms are distinguished from generalized forms:

❖ <u>Barber's palmoplantar pustular psoriasis</u>
Most frequently, favored by smoking, the palmo-plantar involvement is symmetrical, evolving towards erythematosquamous placards, with a trichophytoidea appearance.

❖ <u>Acral pustular psoriasis (acrodermatitis of Hallopeau)</u>
Would be a variant of the previous form with a different topography. Indeed, the involvement is peri-ungual with respect to the palms and soles, with sub-ungual hyperkeratosis, the evolution can be towards a generalization of the lesions with bone resorption.

❖ <u>Generalized pustular psoriasis of von Zumbusch</u>
Severe form, with important general signs, it passes by 3 evolutionary stages:

o *Erythematous phase:* large, bright red, edematous ± scaly erythematous plaques, which may evolve into erythroderma with respect to the palms, soles and face.

o *Pustular phase:* rapid appearance of small yellowish-white, non-follicular pustules covered by a very thin membrane.

o *desquamative phase*: drying of the pustules with a desquamation in large flakes.

The introduction of retinoids has significantly improved its prognosis.

❖ <u>**Bloch-Lapierre pustular psoriasis annulus:**</u>

Can be localized or generalized, it starts with erythematous rings, covered with scales on their internal part and dotted with pustules on their external part. They evolve in an eccentric way
as a centrifugal erythema annulare. [22]

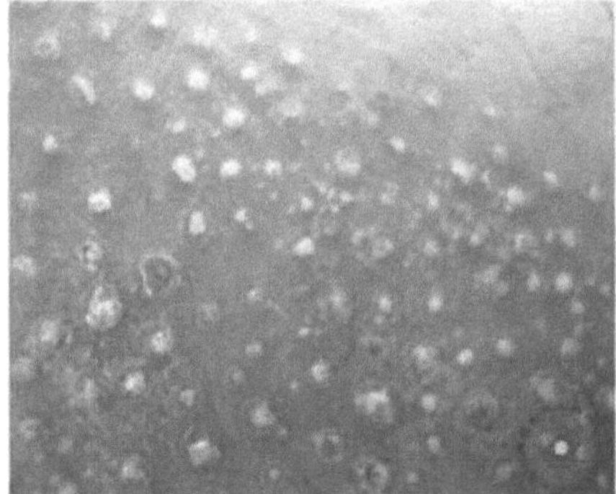

Figure 7: Pustular psoriasis

1.3.8 Psoriatic erythroderma

There are two aspects:

• The dry form: The lesions are generalized, not infiltrated, diffuse with spaces of healthy skin. Scales are less adherent. Pruritus is generally absent. The evolution is good under treatment.

• The wet form: more severe, with generalized erythema and edema, without spaces of healthy skin. Pruritus is important. The general condition is altered with risk of complications and death. [6,16]

In our series, psoriatic erythroderma was present in 3 patients (6.5%).

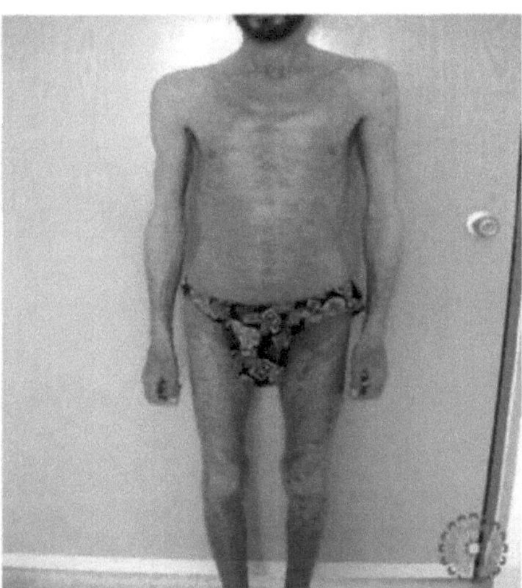

Figure 8: Psoriatic erythroderma

1.3.9 Arthropathic psoriasis :

It is a chronic inflammatory rheumatism, which appears several years after the cutaneous attack and this in two thirds of the cases, one distinguishes the axial form which is more frequent in men, whereas the peripheral attack is seen primarily in women. Joint deformities are possible.

In Morocco, 10% of psoriatic patients develop joint involvement, the average age of onset is between 50 and 60 years with no real gender predominance. [23]

In our study, arthropathic psoriasis accounted for 13%.

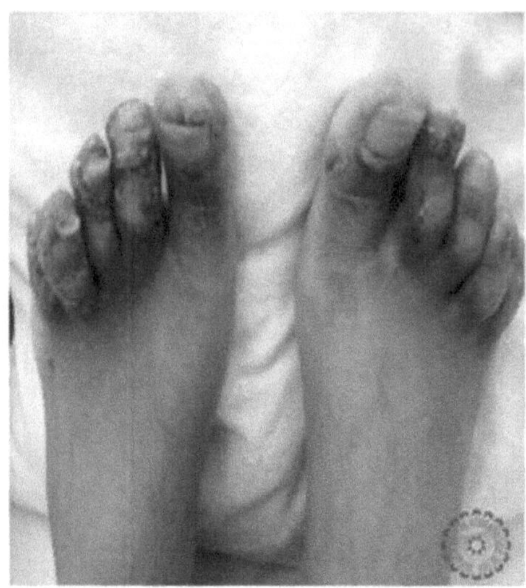

Figure9: Toe deformities in a patient with arthropathic psoriasis with skin manifestations.

1.4 metabolic syndrome :

The metabolic syndrome, also called insulin resistance syndrome, is a group of clinical disorders, frequently associated with psoriasis, including abdominal visceral obesity, insulin resistance, glucose intolerance, hypertension and dyslipidemia. [24,25]

In a study conducted in our department over one year, from November 2011 to November 2012, metabolic syndrome was found in 42% of psoriatic patients.

In the series from the military hospital in Meknes, metabolic syndrome was found in 45%.

1.5   Treatment

The therapeutic arsenal for psoriasis is constantly evolving, especially in terms of biotherapy. The treatment depends on the clinical form but especially on the extent of the lesions.

1.5.1 General measures :

The physician must explain the involvement of genetic and environmental factors in psoriasis, aggravating factors such as stress, infections, especially streptococcal infections, excessive consumption of alcohol and tobacco, as well as the inducing role of certain medications such as beta-blockers, antimalarials, lithium, and interferon

The psychological impact of this chronic pathology, must be taken into consideration by the attending physician, thanks to the DLQI: dermatology index of disease activity (little altered if <5, altered if between 5 and 10, very altered if >10) [26]

1.5.2 Local treatments :

Local treatments are adopted for mild forms of psoriasis, i.e., when the affected body surface area is less than 15% or in combination with other systemic treatments. The main local treatments include dermocorticoids, vitamin D3 analogues, a topical retinoid, salicylic acid, and emollients, which are available in different forms (lotion, ointment) [27]

Tar-based treatments have been abandoned because of the side effects (odors, stains and carcinogenic risks).

❖   <u>Salicylic acid:</u>

Hyperkeratosis reducing treatment, used at concentrations ranging from 2-30% in adults and 1% in children to avoid salicylate intoxication. [27]

❖   <u>Local corticosteroids:</u>

It remains the most widely prescribed treatment for psoriasis with an anti-inflammatory, immunomodulatory and anti-proliferative action on keratinocytes.

They exist with different levels of activity, from low (hydrocortisone) to very high (Betamethasone) and, sometimes combined with other treatments such as salicylic acid (Betamethasone and salicylic acid). This treatment must be of short duration and gradually stopped in order to avoid local side effects such as skin atrophy and tachyphylaxis [28,29].

❖   <u>Vitamin D3 analogues:</u>

Like calcipotriol, they neutralize keratinocyte proliferation and modulate keratinocyte differentiation. They can be associated with a dermocorticoid. Although this treatment does not cause skin atrophy or recurrence after discontinuation of treatment, there is a possibility of skin irritation, especially on the face and folds, and the risk of hypercalcemia and hypoparathyroidism observed especially in patients with renal insufficiency or with calcium metabolism disorders [30].

❖   <u>Topical retinoid (Tazarotene, Zorac ®):</u>

Its use is restricted because of its strong inflammatory and irritating potential (burning, erythema). It acts on hyperproliferation and abnormal differentiation of keratinocytes. [27]

❖   <u>**Sea salt, sulfur and oil baths:**</u>

Can complement local treatments.

1.6   Phototherapy:

The favorable effect of sun exposure on psoriasis is well known. In case of insufficient response to the first type of treatment or in case of more extensive lesions, reaching more than 20% of the body surface, treatment with phototherapy can be considered. The different phototherapy techniques include UVB phototherapy, oral and local Puvatherapy, and natural heliotherapy [27].

J UVB: UVB therapy is often used 2 to 3 times a week with an initial dose depending on the phototype or 70% of the minimal erythema dose with a prudent increase (30% if no erythema, 20% if minimal erythema) once a good response is reached the frequency of treatment should be reduced.

The main side effects: erythema, burning, dyschromia and hyperpigmentation.

Contraindications: xeroderma pigmentosum and other genodermatoses, systemic lupus erythematosus, photodermatoses and skin cancers. [31]

J PUVA-therapy: It combines exposure to UVA radiation (320 to 400nm) at 2 or 3 sessions per week, for about 10 weeks, and the simultaneous use of psoralen, and photo-sensitizing substances such as Meladinin ® or Psoraderm ®. However, it is a second choice because of its numerous contraindications (hypersensitivity to light, cataract, liver and kidney failure), and its adverse effects (pain, allergy, aging and skin cancers). [31]

1.7   Systemic treatments:

For more severe and treatment-resistant forms, systemic therapy with retinoids, methotrexate or cyclosporine is considered [27].

Systemic corticosteroid therapy is prohibited because of the risk of rebound with evolution towards a more severe form such as the pustular or erythrodermic form of psoriasis. For the choice of each treatment, a good knowledge of contraindications and side effects are necessary for a correct administration of these drugs.

<u>**Methotrexate**</u>:

Methotrexate is the subject of our study and will be detailed in another chapter.

<u>**Cyclosporine (Neoral*)**</u>:

Is a potent T-cell specific immunosuppressant that inhibits cell-mediated immune responses. By binding to a specific receptor, it blocks the calcineurin (phosphatase)-dependent activation pathway and consequently inhibits the production of cytokines necessary for the immune response (IL-2) as well as their release. [1, 2, 3, 32, 33,34]

<u>**Retinoids** [Etretinate (Tigason*) Acitretin (Soriatane*)]</u>:

Antimitotic, anti-inflammatory, and immunomodulatory action (action on T lymphocytes, langerhans cells and PNN). They reduce the proliferation of keratinocytes and promote their differentiation. It is teratogenic, hence its contraindication in pregnant women and its mandatory use with contraception during and up to two years after cessation of treatment [1, 2, 3, 34].

<u>**Biological agents**</u>:

In addition to conventional treatments, research on the immune system and its role, particularly that of T cells in psoriasis, has led to the development of biological agents that reduce the extent and severity of the disease and target the underlying causes of psoriasis. They represent an important breakthrough in the treatment of moderate to severe psoriasis.

These biological agents are either fusion proteins or antibodies that inhibit TNF a or lymphocyte activation. They are indicated after failure of 2 systemic treatments including Puvatherapy, or if there is a profound alteration in the quality of life.

Pre-therapeutic workup: infectious workup, antinuclear CA.

Contraindication: progressive infectious pathology; quiescent or evolving tuberculosis; heart failure; cancer or lymphoma; multiple sclerosis; pregnancy or breastfeeding; live attenuated vaccines must be administered before starting treatment. [34-39]

<u>**Etanercept** (Enbrel®)</u>

Is a fully human molecule with a TNF receptor. It is able to bind to TNF, preventing it from reaching its membrane receptors. The binding of etanercept to TNF renders it biologically inactive and thus induces a decrease in inflammatory activity.

❖ Indication: arthropathic psoriasis, rheumatoid arthritis, pustular psoriasis, palmoplantar psoriasis refractory to other treatments. [34-39]

<u>Infliximab</u> *(Remicade®)*

Is a chimeric monoclonal antibody (human-mouse) that binds to TNFa. It inhibits the production of other proinflammatory cytokines, reducing cell infiltration and eventually keratinocyte proliferation.

❖ Indication: psoriatic arthritis, pustular psoriasis in patients resistant to the usual therapies.

❖ Side effects: infections, lymphoma (non-Hodgkin's lymphoma), induction of lupus erythematosus [31,34-39]

<u>Adalimumab</u> *(Humira®)*

It is a recombinant human monoclonal anti-TNFa antibody. In France, adalimumab was first indicated for the treatment of psoriatic arthritis in 2005, and in January 2008 it was granted marketing authorization for the treatment of psoriasis. [31,34-39]

In our series, no patient was able to benefit from biotherapy, because its price is too high compared to the socioeconomic level of our sample, and also because this therapy is not reimbursable in this indication by the health insurance.

2. Methotrexate

Since 1953, methotrexate has been used in the United States as an antineoplastic treatment. And since the 1980s, given its antiproliferative and immunosuppressive properties, methotrexate has been used to treat ectopic pregnancies, but also inflammatory pathologies such as rheumatoid arthritis and psoriasis. [40]

2.1 Mode of action

Methotrexate is an analogue of folic acid, an essential cofactor in the synthesis of deoxyribonucleic acid (DNA) and ribonucleic acid (RNA) precursors. To be active, folic acid must be reduced to tetrahydrofolates by an enzyme called dihydrofolate reductase (DHFR). Methotrexate inhibits DHFR by competing with folic acid, interrupting DNA and RNA synthesis. Thus, it is primarily toxic to rapidly renewing tissues such as intestinal epithelium, bone marrow and neoplastic tissues [40, 41, 42].

[40, 41,42]

2.2 Pharmacodynamic properties

The efficacy of methotrexate in psoriasis results from its antiproliferative action related to the inhibition of DHFR, but also from its anti-inflammatory and immunomodulatory activities, in fact, methotrexate inhibits the chemotaxis of the polynuclear cells, inhibits the cutaneous inflammatory reaction induced by the C5a fraction of the complement, and decreases the number of dendritic cells in the epidermis

Methotrexate may also inhibit IL-1 binding to its receptors on T cells in a dose-dependent manner.

Pharmacokinetics

Absorption

The bioavailability of methotrexate after oral or intramuscular administration at the doses used in dermatology is good. It is approximately 80%. The maximum plasma concentration is reached on average around two hours after oral administration and one hour after intramuscular injection.

Diffusion and protein binding

Methotrexate enters the target cell mainly by an active transport system and a small portion by passive diffusion. It is transformed in the intracellular medium into active polyglutamate derivatives. These derivatives are very slowly released into the extracellular medium and are responsible for the persistent effects of the molecule.

Methotrexate is 50 to 70% bound to plasma proteins, mainly albumin. The free fraction, which is the only active fraction, is increased in the event of hypoalbuminemia or competition with other molecules, thus increasing the risk of toxicity.

Metabolism and elimination

Methotrexate is poorly metabolized by hepatic aldehyde oxidase, the major metabolite being 7-hydroxy-methotrexate. Methotrexate is rapidly eliminated unchanged via the urine (50-80%) and to a lesser extent via the bile duct. It is subject to enterohepatic cycling, which accounts for a prolonged elimination half-life of about ten hours. Elimination is reduced in cases of renal insufficiency, with a risk of increased toxicity of the molecule.

<u>**Concentration-effect relationship**</u>

It has been shown that there is a good correlation between plasma or intra-erythrocyte concentrations of methotrexate and its efficacy on psoriasis lesions. This will allow us to adapt the dosage of the molecule to each patient according to the concentrations measured after the first doses.

<u>**Presentation, route of administration and price**</u>

Methotrexate is administered once a week intramuscularly (Methoject®, Ledertrexate®) or orally (Novatrex®, Imeth®, Méthotrexate Bellon®, Méthotrexate Mylan®, Méthotrexate Teva®). The latter is divided into three doses taken 12 hours apart.

In Morocco, we have the injectable route alone.

Trade name	Active substance	Form & Presentation	Public price Morocco (PPM)	(P) princeps : (G) generic	Reimbursem :ent
LEDERTREXATE	METHOTREXATE 5mg	INJECTABLE SOLUTION (1 bottle 2ml)	20,40 DH	P	REIMBURSEMENT
LEDERTREXATE	METHOTREXATE 25mg	INJECTABLE SOLUTION (1 vial 1ml)	36,30 DH	P	REIMBURSEMENT
METHOTREXAT EBELLON	METHOTREXATE 5mg	INJECTABLE SOLUTION (1 bottle 2ml)	21,20 DH	P	REIMBURSEMENT
METHOTREXAT EBELLON	METHOTREXATE 25mg	INJECTABLE SOLUTION (1 vial 1ml)	36,30 DH	P	REFUNDABLE
METHOTREXAT EMYLAN	METHOTREXATE 5mg	INJECTABLE SOLUTION (10 vials 2ml)	178,00 DH	G	REIMBURSEMENT

<u>**Drug interactions**</u>

There are drug interactions whose mechanisms are the following:

\-   Increased plasma free fraction: this is the case for sulfonamides, salicylic acid, tetracycline, chloramphenicol, phenytoin, phenylbutazone and barbiturates.

\-   Decreased renal elimination: by drugs that reduce renal blood flow such as non-steroidal anti-inflammatory drugs, all nephrotoxic substances, and aspirin.

\-   Decreased digestive absorption: by antibiotics not absorbed by the digestive mucosa such as neomycin or colistin.

\-   Pharmacodynamic interactions: Drugs that decrease intracellular folate levels (sulfonamides, phenytoin) may increase methotrexate toxicity.

Folinic acid is likely to decrease the toxicity and efficacy of methotrexate, whereas folic acid would decrease the toxicity without affecting the efficacy of methotrexate. [40-43]

2.3   *Indication in dermatology*

Methotrexate has the MA, obtained in 1992, for the treatment of psoriasis. The official framework for prescription is "adult psoriasis in its extensive form (more than 50% of the body surface) and resistant to conventional therapies such as puvatherapy and retinoids, psoriatic erythroderma, and generalized pustular psoriasis" [7]. Despite the absence of an official framework until 1992, methotrexate had been used "off-label" for over 30 years by dermatologists in the treatment of psoriasis.

The dosages used in this indication vary from 7.5 to 30 mg/week, seeking as soon as possible the minimal effective dose, taken per os or intramuscularly, in a single weekly dose.

Methotrexate in moderate doses has been used for its anti-inflammatory and or immunosuppressive properties in many other dermatological diseases such as :

❖   Pityriasis rubra pilaris

❖   Cutaneous T-cell lymphomas

❖   Dermatomyositis

❖   Sarcoidosis

❖   Lupus erythematosus ....

Side effects

The main side effects are summarized in the following table:

More **frequent**	**Nausea, malaise, hair loss**
Common	**Transaminase and CBC abnormalities, gastrointestinal ulcers**
Occasional	**Fever, depression, infections**
Rare	**Nephrotoxicity, hepatic fibrosis, cirrhosis**
Very rare	**Interstitial pneumonia, alveolitis**

2.4 Prescription of methotrexate

2.4.1 Pre-therapy assessment

Begins with a thorough clinical examination to look for any contraindications or precautions. The modalities of the treatment must be precisely explained and understood. Effective contraception must be instituted in the woman.

The paraclinical workup consists of a CBC and platelet count, plasma creatinine and urea, transaminases, y-GT, alkaline phosphatases, bilirubin, albuminemia, hepatitis B and C and HIV serologies, pregnancy test, IDR and BK research in the sputum in our Moroccan context with a chest X-ray A pre-therapeutic liver biopsy or a fibroscann should be performed. [40-43]

<u>**Contrary indications absolute**</u>

- Severe infections
- Progressive liver damage and cirrhosis
- Renal insufficiency
- Pregnancy and breastfeeding
- Excessive alcohol consumption
- Hematological damage (anemia, leuko-neutropenia, thrombocytopenia)
- An immune deficiency
- Gastric ulcer
- Respiratory disease

<u>**Other relative indications**</u>

- Hepatic and renal insufficiency
- Advanced age
- Duodenal ulcer
- Viral hepatitis
- Poor compliance with medication
- Desire of pregnancy
- Gastritis
- Diabetes mellitus
- Previous neoplasia
- Congestive heart failure [40-43]

2.4.2 Precaution of administration and association

An initial dose of 5 mg is administered in order to search for an idiosyncratic, non-dose-dependent reaction. Thereafter, if well tolerated, the therapeutic dose will be increased, generally between 7.5 and 30 mg/kg/day, in search of the minimum effective dose. Systematic oral administration of folic acid (Speciafoldine®, 5 mg tablets) at a rate of one tablet per day, except on the day the methotrexate is taken, or at a rate of 2 tablets the day after the injection, makes it possible to significantly improve hematological and digestive tolerance. [44]

2.4.3 Monitoring

CBC and transaminases should be monitored weekly for the first month of treatment, then monthly for the next three months and then once every three months thereafter. Other liver function parameters such as alkaline phosphatases, y-GT and bilirubin, renal function and albumin levels should be monitored every three to six months. An annual chest x-ray should be discussed because of the low risk of progressive fibrosis. In the absence of hepatic abnormalities, a systematic PBH or a fibroscan should be considered for a cumulative dose of between 1.5 and 4 g of methotrexate [40-43]. [40-43]

3. Methotrexate and Psoriasis

3.1 Indication

Methotrexate (MTX) has been the mainstay of treatment for moderate to severe psoriasis since it was first used nearly half a century ago. Over the years, its efficacy, low cost, and relative ease of administration have helped make MTX the drug of choice in the management of moderate to severe psoriasis.

3.2 Efficiency

A study conducted in the Dermatology Department of Casablanca over a period of 15 years (January 1991-December 2004), 2013 patients with psoriasis were collected in the department, including 458 patients hospitalized for severe forms. Among the 458 patients, 77 cases (16.8%) were treated with methotrexate. The weekly dose of methotrexate varied from 10 to 25 mg IM. The average duration of treatment was 78 months. Progression was favorable in 53.2% of cases, with partial remission in 22%. Worsening was noted in 16.8% of cases. [45]

Another study conducted in Tunisia, from January 2002 to December 2009. Twenty-one patients with severe psoriasis who were put on methotrexate were identified. Remission was complete in 62% of cases and partial in 28.5% of cases. [46]

In our series, MTX was necessary after failure of dermocorticoids in 39 cases, calcipotriol in 5 cases and phototherapy in 2 cases. The weekly dose of MTX varied from 10 to 30 mg. The average duration of treatment was 16.19 months. Patients were followed up with a biological check-up (CBC, liver and kidney function tests) and a fibroscann to look for hepatic fibrosis. Folic acid supplementation was performed in 82.7% of patients.

Its efficacy was noted from the third month, 50% of patients were in complete remission after 24 months of treatment. Side effects were rarely encountered in our study, probably due to regular monitoring of patients and folic acid supplementation. In addition, the low price of MTX has broadened the indications for its prescription, especially in patients with a low socioeconomic level. Indeed, the calculation of the cost of treatment over one year for a patient of 60 KG, without taking into account the cost of the check-up, by comparing Remicade and MTX, has resulted in a price of 205752 DH against 1815 DH respectively. MTX remains for us a treatment of choice, which we are used to prescribing: it is safe, effective, low cost and well tolerated. Biotherapies are as effective as MTX with fewer side effects, however their cost remains high, especially since they are not reimbursed by social security. In our context, MTX remains the first-line treatment for moderate to severe psoriasis.

VI.   <u>Limitations of the study</u>

The practical implications of our results, however, are qualified by a number of limitations:

J The retrospective nature of the study posed the problem of collecting data on SKINDEX, nail and scalp involvement.

J Unexpected breaks in MTX, unavailability of the oral form and folic acid, hampered our prescription.

J The need for MTX monitoring checkups, and comorbidities, was sometimes a cause for discontinuation and change of treatment.

VII. <u>Perspectives</u>

We consider the results of our work to be preliminary and in need of further substantiation in the future by large, comparative, multicenter prospective studies with a more representative sample, using validated assessment scores (SKINDEX, DLQI). To compare the efficacy of MTX in the treatment of other dermatoses (dermatomyositis, sarcoidosis, prurigo, pelade,   ) with its efficacy in the treatment of psoriasis.

VIII.   <u>Conclusion</u>

MTX has been the standard treatment for moderate to severe psoriasis for over five decades. Its efficacy is indisputable, and it is important to recognize that MTX will continue to be the mainstay of psoriasis treatment, particularly in developing countries, because of its cost-effectiveness.

IX.   <u>Summary</u>

Introduction

Psoriasis is a chronic inflammatory disease and can be treated locally or systemically. Methotrexate (MTX) is among the systemic treatments for moderate to severe psoriasis.

The aim of our study is to evaluate the place of MTX in the treatment of psoriasis in our Moroccan context.

Materials and methods

Retro prospective study conducted in the dermatology department from 2010 to 2014. All cases of psoriasis were included and the records of patients treated with MTX were studied. A pre-established form was completed for each patient specifying the type of psoriasis, indications, prescription modalities, monitoring, evolution and side effects.

Results

Of all the psoriasis cases, 46 met the inclusion criteria. The patients were male in 58.7% of cases, aged between 18 and 45 years in 45.7% of cases and over 45 years in 41.3% of cases, while 13% were children. The clinical forms were distributed as follows: psoriasis vulgaris in 35 cases (76.1%), followed by arthropathic psoriasis in 6 cases (13%), erythrodermic psoriasis in 3 cases (6.5%) and psoriatic palmoplantar keratosis in 2 cases (4.3%).

56.5% had a body surface area (BSA) between 25 and 50%, 21.7% had a BSA between 50 and 70%. 84.8% were previously treated with dermocorticoids. The weekly dose of MTX varied from 10 to 30 mg. The average duration of treatment was 16.19 months. Patients were followed up with a biological check-up (CBC, liver and kidney tests), and a fibroscann to look for hepatic fibrosis.

The evolution was marked by a complete remission in 50% of cases, with a maximum response obtained at 24 months. Side effects were mainly digestive intolerance, cytolysis and renal failure noted in only 3 cases.

Discussion

MTX is a folic acid analogue with antiproliferative, anti-inflammatory and immunomodulatory activity. It has been used for over 40 years in the treatment of moderate to severe psoriasis. In our series, MTX was necessary after failure of dermocorticoids in 39 cases, calcipotriol in 5 cases and phototherapy in 2 cases. Its efficacy was noted from the third month, 50% of patients were in complete remission after 24 months of treatment. The side effects rarely encountered in our study and the low price of MTX have broadened the indications for its prescription.

Biotherapies are as effective as MTX with fewer side effects, however their cost remains high, especially since they are not reimbursed by social security. In our context, MTX remains the first-line treatment for moderate to severe psoriasis.

<u>Conclusion:</u>

MTX is a reference molecule in the treatment of moderate to severe psoriasis, with a better cost/benefit/risk ratio.

XI. <u>References</u>

[1]   Pathirana D, Nast A,Ormerod AD,Reytan N, Saiag P, Smith CH .Systemic Treatment of Psoriasis vulgaris. J Eur Acad Dermatol Venereol. 2010; 24 (12):1458-67

[2]   Paula C,Bachelez H.Treatment of psoriasis in practice for the rheumatologist. Revue du rhumatisme monographies 2011,78 145-51

[3]   Paul C, Gallini A, Maza A, Montaudié H, Sbidian E, Aractingi S. Evidence-based recommendations on conventional systemic treatments in psoriasis: systematic review and expert opinion of a panel of dermatologists. J Eur Acad Dermatol Venereol. 2011, 25 2:2-11

[4]   Basko P,Petronic R. Psoriasis: epidemiology, natural history, and differential diagnosis. Psoriasis: Targets and Therapy 2012:2 67-76

[5]   Sekkat A. situation and prevalence of psoriasis in Morocco .Ann Dermatol Venerol; 2012; 139:3-4.

[6]   Kellati A. Psoriasis and metabolic syndrome: A case control study with prospective data collection. Thesis in Medicine n°079/13. Fez

[7]   Eljamaly J. Psoriasis and methotrexate: effectiveness, tolerance and therapeutic place. Thesis in Medicine n°079/14.Fez

[8]   Prinz JC. New aspects of the pathogenesis of psoriasis. J Dermatol Ges Dtsch. June 2004; 2 (6):448-56.

[9]   Nikhil Y, Braathen Lasse R. Psoriasis vulgaris: from pathogenesis to treatment Forum Med Suisse 2006;6;549-54

[10]   BERARD F, NICOLAS F .Physiopathology of psoriasis Ann Dermatol Venereol 2003;130:837-42

[11]   Jullien D, Solignac M. A new view of psoriasis. Ann Dermatol Venereol. 2010, 137:3-7.

[12]   Boulinguez S. News - Psoriasis. Ann Dermatol Venereo (2011) 138, 1-5

[13]   Jullien D. Pathophysiology of psoriasis. Ann Dermatol Venereo (2012) 139, 68-72

[14]   Jullien D. Psoriasis: a chronic inflammatory systemic disease Ann Dermatol Venereo (2008)135, 296-300

[15]   Charles w et al. Interleukin 17A: toward a new understanding of psoriasis pathogenesis. JAAD july 2014 volume 71 (1) 141-150

[16]   Benchikhi H, Amal S, Hassam B. The severe forms of psoriasis. Ann Dermatol Venereo 2012; 139:19-25

[17]   Mahé E. de Prost Y.Psoriasis in children. Journal of pediatrics and child care 17 (2004) 380-386

[18]   Karabudak Abuaf O, Dogan B. Management of guttate psoriasis in patients with associated streptococcal infection. Psoriasis: Targets and Therapy 2012:2 89-94

[19]   Richard-Lallemand MA. State of the art on scalp psoriasis. Ann Dermatol Venereo (2009), 136, 34-38

[20]   Feldman SR, Fleischer AB, Rebaussin DM, Rapp SR, Bradham DD, Exum ML et al .The economic impact of psoriasis increases with psoriasis severity. J Am Acad Dermatol 1997; 37; 56469

[21]   Cribier B. Psoriasis: rare or unusual forms. Ann Dermatol Venereo (2012) 139, 39-45

[22]   Bachelez H. Pustular psoriasis. Ann Dermatol Venereo (2012) 139, 34-38

[23]   Icen M, Crowson CS, McEvoy MT, Dann FJ, Gabriel SE, Maradit Kermersh . Trends in incidence of adult onset psoriasis over 3 decades: a population based study. J.Am
Acad Dermaol 2009; 60(3)394-401

[24]   Marne Bhat R, Peter Pinto H. Lipid profile in psoriasis patients. Psoriasis: Targets and Therapy 2012:2 77-80

[25]   Pearson K.C. Armstrong A. W. Psoriasis and cardiovascular disease: epidemiology, mechanisms, and clinical implications. Psoriasis: Targets and Therapy 2012:2 1-11

[26]   Xi Tan, Feldman S R, Balkrishnan R. Quality of life issues and measurement in patients
with psoriasis. Psoriasis: Targets and Therapy 2012:2 13-23

[27]   Thivolet J,Nicolas J. Psoriasis from the clinic to the therapy, 1997,5-21,35_101

[28]   Queille-Roussel C, Paul C, Duteil L, et al. The new topical ascomycin derivative
SCZ ASM 981 does not induce skin atrophy when applied to normal skin for 4 weeks:
a randomized, double-blind controlled study. Br J Dermatol 2001; 144: 507-13.

[29]   Reitamo S, Rissanen J, Remitz A, et al. Tacrolimus does not affect collagen
synthesis: results of a single-center randomized trial. J Invest Dermatol 1998; 111: 396-
98

[30]   Rejeski WJ. Mihalko SL. Physical Activity and Quality of Life in Older
Adults. Journal of Gerontology: Biological and Medical Sciences, 2001 56A. 23-35

[31]   Pathirana D, Ormerod AD, Saiag P, Smith C et al. European S3 Guidelines on
the systemic treatment of psoriasis vulgaris. J Eur Acad Dermatol Venereol 2009; 23

[32]   Robert E, Kalb B, Strober P, Gerald W. Methotrexate and psoriasis: 2009
National Psoriasis Foundation Consensus Conference. J AM ACAD DERMATOL 60,
5, 824-837

[33]   Cuellar ML, Espinoza LR. Use of methotrexate in psoriasis and psoriatic
arthritis. Rheum Dis Clin North Am. November 1997; 23 (4):797-809.
[34]   Pathirana D et al. European S3-Guidelines on the systemic treatment of
psoriasis vulgaris. J Eur Acad Dermatol Venereol (2009)

[35]   Levy L, Solomon S M, Emer J J. Biologics in the treatment of psoriasis and
emerging new therapies in the pipeline. Psoriasis: Targets and Therapy 2012:2 29-43

[36]   Molteni S, Reali E. Biomarkers in the pathogenesis, diagnosis, and treatment
of psoriasis Psoriasis: Targets and Therapy 2012:2 55-66

[37]   Kimball A.B. Long-term efficacy and safety of ustekinumab in patients with
moderate-to-severe psoriasis after five years of follow-up. Ann Dermatol Venereo
(2012).10.258

[38]   Levy-Roya A, Porchera R, de Fonclared A L, Morela P, Dupuya A. Efficacy
of anti-TNF agents in psoriasis: a systematic review and graphical representation. Ann
Dermatol Venereo (2009) 136, 315-22

[39]   Viguier M. Efficacy and tolerability of anti-TNF alpha in generalized pustular
psoriasis. Ann Dermatol Venereo (2012) 10.013

[40]   Lebrun-Vignes B, Bachelez H, Chosidow O. Methotrexate in dermatology:

pharmacology, indications, use and precautions. Rev Med Interne 1999; 20: 384-92

[41]   Roenigk HH Jr , Auerbach R , Maibach H , G Weinstein , Lebwohl M . Methotrexate in psoriasis: consensus conference J Am Acad Dermatol. 1998; 38 (3):478-85.

[42]   Montaudie H. Methotrexate in psoriasis: a systematic review of treatment modalities, incidence, risk factors and monitoring of liver toxicity. J Eur Acad Dermatol Venereol 2011, 25:1218

[43]   Beylot-Barrya M, Le Maitre M. Methotrexate. Ann Dermatol Venereo (2011) 138, 833-35

[44]   Psoriasis Research Group of the French Society of Dermatology. Information letter on treatment of psoriasis with methotrexate. Ann Dermatol Venereol. 2011; 138 (12) :874-5

[45]   Skali SS, Jamali Mj, Benchikhi Hb Lakhdar Hl. Psoriasis and methotrexate: 77 cases. Ann Dermatol Venereol 2005;132:971-79

[46]   Khaled A, Ben Hamida M, Zeglaoui F, Kharfi M, Ezzine N, Fazaa B. Treatment of psoriasis by methotrexate in the period of biotherapies: a study in 21 Tunisian patients. Thérapie.2012; 67 (1) :49-52.

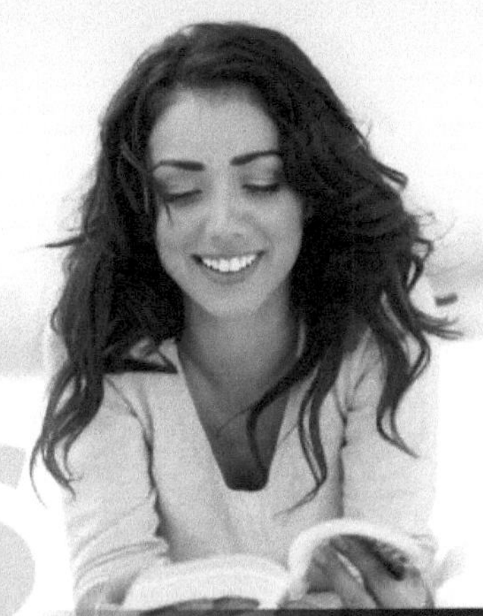

I want morebooks!

Buy your books fast and straightforward online - at one of world's fastest growing online book stores! Environmentally sound due to Print-on-Demand technologies.

Buy your books online at
www.morebooks.shop

Kaufen Sie Ihre Bücher schnell und unkompliziert online – auf einer der am schnellsten wachsenden Buchhandelsplattformen weltweit! Dank Print-On-Demand umwelt- und ressourcenschonend produzi ert.

Bücher schneller online kaufen
www.morebooks.shop

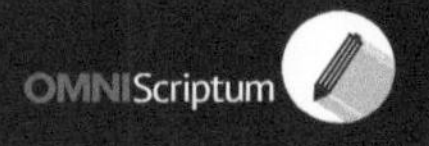

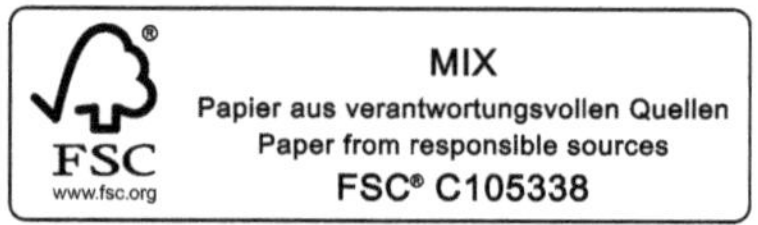

Printed by Books on Demand GmbH, Norderstedt / Germany